Keto
Cookbook
for women after 50

Judith Green

Table of contents

Introduction 7

Chapter 1. Breakfast Recipes.............................19

1   Pork Sausage and Egg Cup......................20

2   Lemon Cake with Poppy Seeds 21

3   Sesame & Poppy Seed Bagels.......................23

4   Mushroom and Egg Cups.............................24

5   Coconut Crepes with Vanilla Cream 25

Chapter 2. Snack & Appetizer Recipes.......................27

6   Bacon Fat Bombs 27

7   Crab Egg Scramble 29

8   Cream Cheese Stuffed Mushrooms.................30

9   Zucchini Chips..31

10   Hot Spare Ribs 32

Chapter 3. Poultry Recipes.......................................35

11   Rosemary Turkey with Celery 35

12   Turkey with Mustard Gravy.........................37

13   Spicy Turkey with Peppers 39

14   Paprika Turkey Breast 41

15   Cheese Chicken Drumsticks in Wine 42

Chapter 4. Beef 45

16   Spicy Beef Brisket Roast 45

17   Caribbean Beef with Peppers........................ 48

18   Veal with Ham and Sauerkraut 49

19   Pepperoni and Beef Pizza Meatloaf............ 50

20   Beef Chuck Roast with Mushrooms 52

Chapter 5. Lamb 53

21   White Wine Lamb Chops............................. 53

22   Oven-Roasted Lamb Chops With Fragrant
Curry Sauce..55

23   Grilled Lamb Chops with Dijon Basil Butter 57

24   Lamb Chops with Tapenade 58

25   Lamb Lollipops With Garlic And Rosemary 60

Chapter 6. Pork Recipes 61

26   Pork and Green Salad 61

27   Cayenne Pork Saag 64

28   Pork Bacon with Mixed Greens 66

29   Pork Cutlets with Mushroom Sauce 67

30   Pork Shank with Radish 69

Chapter 7. Fish and Seafood 71

31   Lemon Butter Scallops................................. 71

32   Mackerel with Bell Pepper........................... 74

33   Dijon Shrimp with Romaine......................... 75

34   Cheese Mussel and Tomato Stew 77

35   Dijon Crab Cake 79

Chapter 8. Vegetable Recipes 81

36   Romano Zucchini Cups 81

37   Pumpkin and Cauliflower Curry 83

38   Garlic Broccoli with Fresh Basil 84

39   Cauliflower Egg Bake 86

40   Zucchini Casserole 87

Chapter 9. Soup Recipes 89

41   Mixed Mushroom Soup 89

42   Broccoli & Fennel Soup 91

43   Keto Reuben Soup 92

44   Effortless Chicken Chili 93

45   Parsnip–Tomato Soup 94

Chapter 10. Dessert Recipes 95

46   Bacon Fudge 95

47   Blueberry Crisp 98

48   Lemon Coconut Balls 99

49   Almond Shortbread Cookies 101

50   Granny Smith Apple Tart 103

Why Is It Important for People Over 50?

As you grow in age, the body's natural fat-burning ability reduces. When that happens, your body stops receiving a healthy dose of nutrients properly, which is why you will develop diseases and ailments. With the keto diet, you are pushing the body into ketosis and bypassing the need to worry about your body's ability to burn fat. Once in ketosis, your body will now burn fat forcefully for survival.

Once more, your system will now start to regain strength. An even better aspect that follows is your insulin level because it drops. If you are someone diagnosed with diseases such as type 2 diabetes and others, the drop in insulin might even reverse the effects and eliminate the diseases from your body altogether.

There are studies underway, and most of them suggest that the keto diet is far more beneficial to those above 50 than it is for those under this age bracket. A quick search on Google and you are immediately overwhelmed with over 93 million results, most of which explain the benefits of the keto diet for people above 50. That is a staggering number for a diet plan that has only been around a few years.

It is also important to highlight that as we get older, we start losing more than just the ability to burn fat. During this phase of our life, once we hit around 50 years of age, we come across various obstacles, some chronic in nature, which transpire only because our body is no longer able to function at rates like it did when we were young. Ketogenic diets help us regain that edge and feel energized from within.

There are hundreds of thousands of stories, all pointing out how this revolutionary diet is especially helpful for older adults and the elderly. It is, therefore, a no-brainer for people above 50 who have spent ages trying to search for a healthy lifestyle choice of diet. With such a high success rate, there is no harm in trying, right?

Before the keto phenomenon, there was the Atkins diet. The Atkins diet was also a low-carb diet, just like its keto counterpart. This form of diet also became a huge hit with the masses. However, unlike keto, the Atkins diet provided weight loss while putting a person through constant hunger. Keto, on the other hand, takes away that element, and it does that using ketosis. Constant exposure to ketosis reduces appetite, hence taking away the biggest hurdle in most diets. The Atkins diet failed to address that front, which is why it was more of a hit and miss. However, credit where it is due, the Atkins diet did garner quite a bit of fame.

However, since the inception of keto, things have changed dramatically.

A study was conducted where 34 overweight adults were monitored and observed for 12 months. All of them were put on keto diets. The result showed that participants had lower HgbA1c (hemoglobin A1c) levels, experienced significant weight loss, and were more likely to completely discontinue their medications for diabetes.

All in all, the keto diet is shaping up to be quite a promising candidate for older adults. Not only will this diet allow us to lead a healthier lifestyle, but it will also curb our ailments and ensure high energy around the clock. That is quite the resume for a diet and one that now seems too attractive to pass up. This is the point where I made up my mind and decided to give the keto diet a go, and I recommend the same to you.

Whether you are a man or a woman, if you have put on weight, or you are suffering from ailments like type 2 diabetes, consider this as your ticket to a care-free world where you will lead a healthy life and rise out of the ailments eventually.

Keto has been producing results that have attracted the top minds and researchers for a fairly long time. Considering the unique nature of this lifestyle of eating, the results have been rather encouraging.

"Great! How do I start?"

Not so fast. While the keto diet is simple, there are a few things I should point out which you should know. Some of these might even change your mind about the entire keto diet plan, but if you are determined for a healthy lifestyle and a fit body, I assure you these should not be of much trouble.

Preparing Yourself for Keto

When entering the world of keto, quite a few of us just pick up a recipe on the internet and start cooking things accordingly. While that is good, we do tend to search for any specifics which we should know of, such as what would happen if I replace nuts with something else? Is oatmeal a part of the keto diet? What are keto-approved food items? Are there any risks involved?

Here is some more information regarding such questions:

· Keto is an extremely strict food diet where you can only eat things that can be classified as keto worthy. Anything that falls out of this category is a straight "no!"

· Keto is a completely new lifestyle. That means your body will undergo some changes. While most of these will be good, some may pose problems such as the keto flu. Most of the people I know, including myself, faced this "flu" with similar symptoms to influenza. It was only after some research that I realized this was natural. The keto flu isn't exactly alarming, but it is best to be mentally prepared for it.

· You will need to work on your cooking skills as keto strictly pushes processed, high-carb foods out of the diet.

· If you aren't really into the idea of protein and fat intake, you may wish to reconsider as these are the two primary areas keto focuses on.

· Apart from this, there are some mistakes people tend to make when they begin their journey. Some of the most common mistakes are:

· Not knowing the keto food properly: Just because something looks like a keto-friendly item doesn't mean it is keto-approved. Always refer to some food guide to check if the item you are interested in is a part of the "good food" in keto.

· Keeping the same level of fat intake throughout: This often leads to results that show in the start and then disappear. You need to constantly adjust your diet and monitor your protein and fat intake.

· Consuming bullet-proof coffee when you really shouldn't: This coffee involves a mixture of coconut oil and butter within coffee. While it is a perfect way to keep hunger at bay, it does push the level of bad cholesterol upwards. If you are someone who has been advised to stick to lower cholesterol levels and avoid consuming similar food items, keep this one off the limits.

· Thinking the keto flu is the only issue to face: Other difficulties will emerge within the first 10 weeks of your keto journey. This will include lethargic limbs, which will make walking difficult at first. Owing to the change in fiber intake, you may either face diarrhea or constipation as well.

· Pushing bodies with vigorous exercises: You have just started keto, give your body a bit of time to adjust. Keep things slow and steady.

· Not replenishing electrolytes: Since we mentioned diarrhea and exercise, your body will run low on electrolytes faster than usual. This is something that you may want to keep in check. Think of sodium and potassium!

These are some of the most common mistakes people have made, and surprisingly, even I was no exception. If only I had someone to properly guide me back then.

Now then, you know the "what" and the "how" of keto, but you are yet to figure out whether this diet is meant for women or men. As a part of the first step, I will now provide you more details regarding both aspects and give you a breakdown of facts to show just how beneficial this diet is for both.

Allowed Product List

If you've decided to go on Keto after 50, be sure you won't regret your choice! So when you start something new, the first and the main thing you need to do is consult the Keto dietary features. But most importantly, you must look at the list of allowed products to remember this list and adhere strictly to it. Don't worry! The low-carb eating plan isn't overly limited. Check out what products you can and must buy in the supermarket and start a new phase in your life.

Meat and Poultry

Chicken, beef, pork, lamb, turkey, veal include no-carb, but high protein and fat intake. That is the primary reason why meat and poultry products are known as staples for the Ketogenic diet. Besides this, bacon and organ meats are also allowed for consumption.

Seafood

When it comes to seafood, you also have an excellent list. You can buy and cook a lot of delicious dishes from:
· Lobster
· Shrimp

- Octopus
- Salmon
- Tuna
- Oysters
- Mussels
- Squid
- Scallops

The most useful Keto seafood is crab and shrimp. They don't contain carbohydrates at all.

Vegetables

Only low-carb and non-starchy veggies can be eaten by the people who go on the Keto diet. This means that you can add the following vegetables:

- Avocados
- Tomatoes
- Cucumbers
- Zucchini
- Radishes
- Mushrooms
- Eggplant
- Celery
- Bell peppers
- Herbs
- Asparagus
- Kohlrabi

- Mustard
- Spinach
- Lettuce
- Kale
- Brussel sprouts

Dairy Products

You should be careful with dairy. Not all dairy food can be useful for you if you want to stick to the Keto diet. Here are the products you can buy and cook:

- Eggs
- Butter and ghee
- Heavy cream and whipping cream
- Sour cream
- Unflavored Greek yogurt
- Cottage cheese
- Hard, semi-hard, soft, and cream cheeses

Berries

Unfortunately, most fruits have high levels of carbs and can't be included in the Keto diet. However, you can consume:

- Blackberries
- Raspberries
- Strawberries
- Blueberries

Nuts and Seeds

A lot of experts recommend paying attention to nuts and seeds that are high-fat and low-carb. You can add such nuts and seeds to your dishes as:

· Almond
· Pecans
· Walnuts
· Hazelnuts
· Brazil nuts
· Pumpkin seeds
· Sesame seeds
· Chia seeds
· Flaxseed

Coconut and Olive Oils

To cook tasty fatty dishes, you need oil. Coconut and olive oils have unique properties that make them suitable for a Keto diet. These oils are rich in fat and boost ketone production. Moreover, they can be used for salad dressing and adding to cooked dishes.

Low-Carb Drinks

The Keto diet means that you should drink only unsweetened coffee and tea because they don't include carbs and fasten metabolism. Besides, you can drink dark chocolate and cocoa. Such drinks have low levels of carbohydrates, and that's why they're permitted.

Prohibited Product List

When it comes to the lists of foods you should avoid on the low-carb, high-fat diet, be attentive and check it carefully. Well, you can't eat:

· Grains (like oatmeal, pasta, bulgur, corn, wheat, buckwheat, rice, etc.)

· Low-fat dairy (fat-free yogurt, skim milk, skim Mozzarella, etc.)

· Most fruits (melon, watermelon, apples, peaches, bananas, grapes, oranges, plums, grapefruits, mangos, cherries, pineapples, pears, etc.)

· Starchy veggies (potatoes, beets, turnips, parsnips, etc.)

· Grain foods (pasta, popcorn, muesli, cereal, bagels, bread, etc.)

· Some oils (soybean oil, grapeseed oil, sunflower oil, peanut oil, canola oil)

· Typical snack foods (crackers, potato chips, etc.)

· Trans fats (margarine.)

· Sweets (candies, buns, pastries, cakes, chocolate, puddings, cookies.)

· Sweeteners and added sugars (corn syrup, cane sugar, honey, agave nectar, etc.)

- Sweetened drinks (sweetened coffee and tea, juice, soda, smoothies.)
- Alcohol (sweet wines, cider, beer, etc.)

Chapter 1. Breakfast Recipes

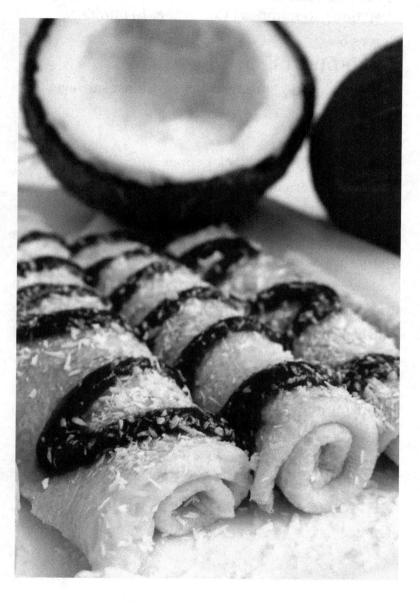

1   Pork Sausage and Egg Cup

Prep time: 10 minutes | Cook time: 15 minutes | Serves 6

INGREDIENTS:

12 ounces (340 g) ground pork breakfast sausage

6 large eggs

½ teaspoon salt

¼ teaspoon ground black pepper

½ teaspoon crushed red pepper flakes

DIRECTIONS:

Place sausage in six 4-inch ramekins (about 2 ounces (57 g) per ramekin) greased with cooking oil. Press sausage down to cover bottom and about ½-inch up the sides of ramekins. Crack one egg into each ramekin and sprinkle evenly with salt, black pepper, and red pepper flakes.

Place ramekins into air fryer basket. Adjust the temperature to 350°F (180°C) and set the timer for 15 minutes. Egg cups will be done when sausage is fully cooked to at least 145°F (63°C) and the egg is firm. Serve warm.

NUTRITION: Cal: 267 | fat: 21g | protein: 14g | carbs: 1g | net carbs: 1g | fiber: 0g

2 Lemon Cake with Poppy Seeds

Prep time: 10 minutes | Cook time: 14 minutes |
Serves 6

INGREDIENTS:

1 cup blanched finely ground almond flour

½ cup powdered erythritol

½ teaspoon baking powder

¼ cup unsalted butter, melted

¼ cup unsweetened almond milk

2 large eggs

1 teaspoon vanilla extract

1 medium lemon

1 teaspoon poppy seeds

DIRECTIONS:

In a large bowl, mix almond flour, erythritol, baking powder, butter, almond milk, eggs, and vanilla.

Slice the lemon in half and squeeze the juice into a small bowl, then add to the batter.

Using a fine grater, zest the lemon and add 1 tablespoon zest to the batter and stir. Add poppy seeds to batter.

Pour batter into nonstick 6-inch round cake pan. Place pan into the air fryer basket.

Adjust the temperature to 300°F (150°C) and set the timer for 14 minutes.

When fully cooked, a toothpick inserted in center will come out mostly clean. The cake will finish cooking and firm up as it cools. Serve at room temperature.

NUTRITION: Cal: 204 | fat: 18g | protein: 6g | carbs: 17g | net carbs: 15g | fiber: 2g

3   Sesame & Poppy Seed Bagels

Total Time: approx. 25 minutes | 4 servings

INGREDIENTS:

½ cup coconut flour

6 eggs

½ cup water

½ cup flax seed meal

½ tsp onion powder

½ tsp garlic powder

1 tsp dried oregano

1 tsp sesame seeds

1 tsp poppy seeds

DIRECTIONS:

Mix the coconut flour, eggs, water, flax seed meal, onion powder, garlic powder, and oregano.

Spoon the mixture into a greased donut tray.

Sprinkle with poppy seeds and sesame seeds.

Bake the bagels for 20 minutes at 360 F.

Let cool on a wire rack for 5 minutes before serving.

NUTRITION: Cal 431; Fat 20g; Net Carbs 1.3g; Protein 29g

4   Mushroom and Egg Cups

Prep time: 10 minutes | Cook time: 7 to 8 minutes | Serves 4

INGREDIENTS:

4 eggs, beaten

1 cup diced mushrooms

½ cup grated sharp Cheddar cheese

¼ cup heavy cream

1 teaspoon salt

1 teaspoon freshly ground black pepper

2 tablespoons chopped fresh cilantro

DIRECTIONS:

In a medium bowl, stir together all the ingredients. Divide the mixture among four glass jars. Place the lids on top of the jars, but do not tighten.

Pour 2 cups water and insert the trivet in the Instant Pot. Place the egg jars on the trivet.

Set the lid in place. Select the Manual mode and set the cooking time for 5 minutes on High Pressure. When the timer goes off, do a quick pressure release. Carefully open the lid.

Remove the jars from the pot and remove the lids from the jars. Serve warm.

NUTRITION: Cal: 238 | fat: 16.8g | protein: 15.1g | carbs: 6.7g | net carbs: 4.7g | fiber: 2.0g

5 Coconut Crepes with Vanilla Cream

Total Time: approx. 35 minutes | 4 servings

INGREDIENTS:

2 tbsp unsweetened cocoa powder

2 cups coconut flour

6 eggs

2 cups flax milk

1 tbsp coconut oil, melted

Vanilla cream

¼ cup butter

2 tbsp erythritol

½ tsp vanilla extract

½ cup coconut cream

DIRECTIONS:

Beat the eggs with a whisk in a bowl.

Add the coconut flour, cocoa powder, baking powder, flax milk, and coconut oil and mix until well combined.

Set a skillet over medium heat, grease with cooking spray, and pour in a ladleful of the batter.

Swirl the pan quickly to spread the dough around the skillet and cook the crepe for 2-3 minutes.

Slide the crepe into a flat plate.

Continue cooking until the remaining batter has finished.

Put the butter and erythritol in a saucepan and melt the butter over medium heat while stirring continuously.

Stir in the coconut cream, reduce the heat to low, and let the sauce simmer for 6-8 minutes while stirring continually.

Turn the heat off and stir in the vanilla extract.

Once the crepes are ready, drizzle the sauce over them, and serve.

NUTRITION: Cal 326; Fat 22g; Net Carbs 5.1g; Protein 10g

Chapter 2. Snack & Appetizer Recipes

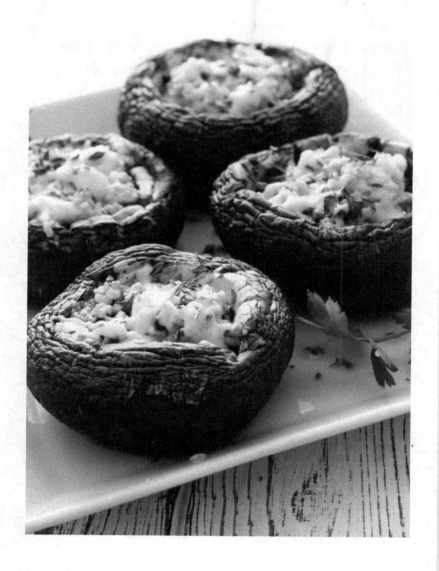

6   Bacon Fat Bombs

Prep time: 15 minutes | Cook time: 0 minutes |
Serves 8

INGREDIENTS:

½ stick butter, at room temperature

8 ounces (227 g) cottage cheese, at room temperature

8 ounces (227 g) Mozzarella cheese, crumbled

1 teaspoon shallot powder

1 teaspoon Italian seasoning blend

2 ounces (57 g) bacon bits

DIRECTIONS:

Mix the butter, cheese, shallot powder, and Italian seasoning blend until well combined.

Place the mixture in your refrigerator for about 60 minutes.

Shape the mixture into 18 balls. Roll each ball in the bacon bits until coated on all sides. Enjoy!

NUTRITION:

calories: 150 | fat: 9.4g | protein: 13.0g | carbs: 2.1g | net carbs: 1.6g | fiber: 0.5g

7 Crab Egg Scramble

Prep time: 15 minutes | Cook time: 0 minutes |
Serves 4

INGREDIENTS:

1 tablespoon olive oil

8 eggs

6 ounces (170 g) crabmeat

Salt and black pepper to taste

Sauce:

¾ cup crème fraiche

½ cup chives, chopped

½ teaspoon garlic powder

Salt to taste

DIRECTIONS:

Whisk the eggs with a fork in a bowl, and season with salt and black pepper.

Set a sauté pan over medium heat and warm olive oil. Add in the eggs and scramble them.

Stir in crabmeat and cook until cooked thoroughly. In a mixing dish, combine crème fraiche and garlic powder. Season with salt and sprinkle with chives. Serve the eggs with the white sauce.

NUTRITION:

calories: 406 | fat: 32.6g | protein: 23.3g | carbs: 4.3g | net carbs: 4.2g | fiber: 0.1g

8   Cream Cheese Stuffed Mushrooms

Prep time: 15 minutes | Cook time: 40 minutes | Serves 10

INGREDIENTS:

20 button mushrooms, stalks removed

6 ounces (170 g) cream cheese

¼ cup mayonnaise

¼ teaspoon mustard seeds

½ teaspoon celery seeds

Sea salt and black pepper, to taste

DIRECTIONS:

Adjust an oven rack to the center position. Brush your mushrooms with nonstick cooking spray and arrange them on a baking sheet.

Roast your mushrooms in the preheated oven at 375°F (190°C) for 40 minutes until the mushrooms release liquid.

In the meantime, mix the remaining ingredients until well combined. Spoon the mixture into the roasted mushroom caps. Bon appétit!

NUTRITION:

calories: 104 | fat: 9.8g | protein: 2.6g | carbs: 2.0g | net carbs: 1.5g | fiber: 0.5g

9 Zucchini Chips

Prep time: 10 minutes | Cook time: 20 minutes |
Serves 2

INGREDIENTS:

1 tablespoon extra-virgin olive oil

¼ teaspoon sea salt

1 teaspoon hot paprika

½ pound (227 g) zucchini, sliced into rounds

2 tablespoons Parmesan cheese, grated

DIRECTIONS:

Gently toss the sliced zucchini with the olive oil, salt,
and paprika. Place them on a tinfoillined baking sheet.
Sprinkle the Parmesan cheese evenly over each
zucchini round.

Bake in the preheated oven at 400°F (205°C) for 15 to
20 minutes or until your chips turns a golden-brown
color.

NUTRITION:

calories: 53 | fat: 4.5g | protein: 1.6g | carbs: 1.5g | net
carbs: 0.9g | fiber: 0.6g

10   Hot Spare Ribs

Prep time: 20 minutes | Cook time: 2 hours | Serves 2

INGREDIENTS:

1 pound (454 g) spare ribs

1 teaspoon Dijon mustard

1 tablespoon rice wine

Salt and ground black pepper, to season

1 teaspoon garlic, pressed

½ shallot powder

1 teaspoon cayenne pepper

½ teaspoon ground allspice

1 tablespoon avocado oil

Hot Sauce:

1 teaspoon Sriracha sauce

1 tablespoon olive oil

1 cup tomato sauce, sugar-free

1 teaspoon garlic, minced

Salt, to season

DIRECTIONS:

Arrange the spare ribs on a parchment-lined baking pan. Add the remaining ingredients for the ribs and toss until well coated.

Bake in the preheated oven at 360°F (182°C) for 1 hour. Rotate the pan and roast an additional 50 to 60 minutes. Baste the ribs with the cooking liquid periodically.

In the meantime, whisk the sauce ingredients until well mixed. Pour the hot sauce over the ribs. Place under the broiler and broil for 7 to 9 minutes or until an internal temperature reaches 145°F (63°C).

Brush the sauce onto each rib and serve warm. Bon appétit!

NUTRITION:

calories: 471 | fat: 27.1g | protein: 48.6g | carbs: 6.6g | net carbs: 4.6g | fiber: 2.0g

Chapter 3. Poultry Recipes

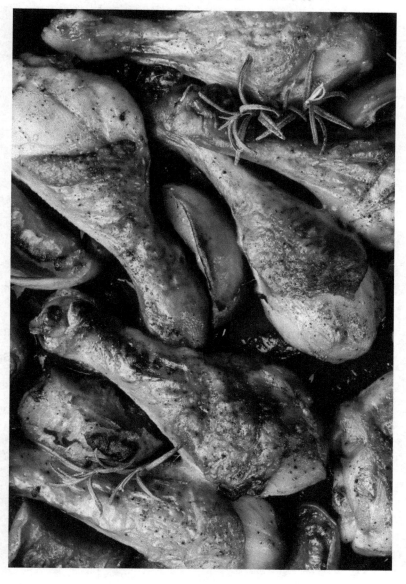

11 Rosemary Turkey with Celery

Prep time: 50 minutes | Cook time: 45 minutes |
Serves 6

INGREDIENTS:

2½ pounds (1.1kg) turkey breasts

1 tablespoon fresh rosemary, chopped

1 teaspoon sea salt

½ teaspoon ground black pepper

1 onion, chopped

1 celery stalk, chopped

DIRECTIONS:

Start by preheating your Air Fryer to 360°F (182°C).
Spritz the sides and bottom of the cooking basket with
a nonstick cooking spray.

Place the turkey in the cooking basket. Add the
rosemary, salt, and black pepper. Cook for 30 minutes
in the preheated Air Fryer.

Add the onion and celery and cook an additional 15
minutes. Bon appétit!

NUTRITION: Cal: 316 | fat: 14g | protein: 41g | carbs:
2g | net carbs: 1g | fiber: 1g

12 Turkey with Mustard Gravy

Prep time: 50 minutes | Cook time: 20 minutes | Serves 6

INGREDIENTS:

2 teaspoons butter, softened

1 teaspoon dried sage

2 sprigs rosemary, chopped

1 teaspoon salt

¼ teaspoon freshly ground black pepper, or more to taste

1 whole turkey breast

2 tablespoons turkey vegetable broth

2 tablespoons whole-grain mustard

1 tablespoon butter

DIRECTIONS:

Start by preheating your Air Fryer to 360°F (182°C).

To make the rub, combine 2 tablespoons of butter, sage, rosemary, salt, and pepper; mix well to combine and spread it evenly over the surface of the turkey breast.

Roast for 20 minutes in an Air Fryer cooking basket. Flip the turkey breast over and cook for a further 15 to 16 minutes. Now, flip it back over and roast for 12 minutes more.

While the turkey is roasting, whisk the other ingredients in a saucepan. After that, spread the gravy all over the turkey breast.

Let the turkey rest for a few minutes before carving. Bon appétit!

NUTRITION: Cal: 384 | fat: 8g | protein: 131g | carbs: 2g | net carbs: 1g | fiber: 1g

13 Spicy Turkey with Peppers

Prep time: 40 minutes | Cook time: 36 minutes | Serves 4

INGREDIENTS:

½ medium-sized leek, chopped

½ red onion, chopped

2 garlic cloves, minced

1 jalapeño pepper, seeded and minced

1 bell pepper, seeded and chopped

2 tablespoons olive oil

1 pound (454 g) ground turkey, 85% lean 15% fat

2 cups tomato purée

2 cups chicken stock

½ teaspoon black peppercorns

Salt, to taste

1 teaspoon chili powder

1 teaspoon mustard seeds

1 teaspoon ground cumin

DIRECTIONS:

Start by preheating your Air Fryer to 365°F (185°C).

Place the leeks, onion, garlic and peppers in a baking pan; drizzle olive oil evenly over the top. Cook for 4 to 6 minutes.

Add the ground turkey. Cook for 6 minutes more or until the meat is no longer pink.

Now, add the tomato purée, 1 cup of chicken stock, black peppercorns, salt, chili powder, mustard seeds, and cumin to the baking pan. Cook for 24 minutes, stirring every 7 to 10 minutes.

Bon appétit!

NUTRITION: Cal: 271 | fat: 15g | protein: 6g | carbs: 11g | net carbs: 10g | fiber: 1g

14 Paprika Turkey Breast

Prep time: 5 minutes | Cook time: 45 to 55 minutes | Serves 10

INGREDIENTS:

1 tablespoon sea salt

1 teaspoon paprika

1 teaspoon onion powder

1 teaspoon garlic powder

½ teaspoon freshly ground black pepper

4 pounds (1.8 kg) bone-in, skin-on turkey breast

2 tablespoons unsalted butter, melted

DIRECTIONS:

In a small bowl, combine the salt, paprika, onion powder, garlic powder, and pepper.

Sprinkle the seasonings all over the turkey. Brush the turkey with some of the melted butter.

Set the air fryer to 350°F (180°C). Place the turkey in the air fryer basket, skin-side down, and cook for 25 minutes.

Flip the turkey and brush it with the remaining butter. Continue cooking for another 20 to 30 minutes, until an instant-read thermometer reads 160°F.

Remove the turkey breast from the air fryer. Tent a piece of aluminum foil over the turkey, and allow it to rest for about 5 minutes before serving.

NUTRITION: Cal: 278 | fat: 14g | protein: 34g | carbs: 2g | net carbs: 1g | fiber: 1g

15   Cheese Chicken Drumsticks in Wine

Prep time: 3 minutes | Cook time: 23 minutes | Serves 5

INGREDIENTS:

1 tablespoon olive oil

5 chicken drumsticks

½ cup chicken stock

¼ cup unsweetened coconut milk

¼ cup dry white wine

2 garlic cloves, minced

1 teaspoon shallot powder

½ teaspoon marjoram

½ teaspoon thyme

6 ounces (170 g) ricotta cheese

4 ounces (113 g) Cheddar cheese

½ teaspoon cayenne pepper

¼ teaspoon ground black pepper

Sea salt, to taste

DIRECTIONS:

Set your Instant Pot to Sauté and heat the olive oil until sizzling.

Add the chicken drumsticks and brown each side for 3 minutes.

Stir in the chicken stock, milk, wine, garlic, shallot powder, marjoram, thyme.

Lock the lid. Select the Manual mode and set the cooking time for 15 minutes at High Pressure.

When the timer beeps, perform a natural pressure release for 10 minutes, then release any remaining pressure. Carefully remove the lid.

Shred the chicken with two forks and return to the Instant Pot.

Set your Instant Pot to Sauté again and add the remaining ingredients and stir well.

Cook for another 2 minutes, or until the cheese is melted. Taste and add more salt, if desired. Serve immediately.

NUTRITION: Cal: 413 | fat: 24.3g | protein: 41.9g | carbs: 4.6g | net carbs: 4.0g | fiber: 0.6g

Chapter 4. Beef

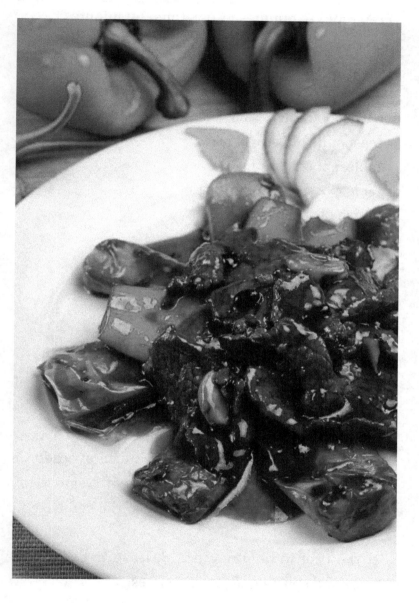

16 Spicy Beef Brisket Roast

Prep time: 15 minutes | Cook time: 60 minutes |
Serves 4

INGREDIENTS:

2 pounds (907 g) beef brisket

½ teaspoon celery salt

1 teaspoon chili powder

1 tablespoon avocado oil

1 tablespoon sweet paprika

A pinch of cayenne pepper

½ teaspoon garlic powder

½ cup beef stock

1 tablespoon garlic, minced

¼ teaspoon dry mustard

DIRECTIONS:

Preheat oven to 340°F (171°C). In a bowl, combine the paprika with dry mustard, chili powder, salt, garlic powder, cayenne pepper, and celery salt. Rub the meat with this mixture.

Set a pan over medium heat and warm avocado oil, place in the beef, and sear until brown. Remove to a baking dish. Pour in the stock, add garlic and bake for 60 minutes.

Set the beef to a cutting board, leave to cool before slicing and splitting in serving plates.

Take the juices from the baking dish and strain, sprinkle over the meat, and enjoy.

NUTRITION:

calories: 481 | fat: 23.6g | protein: 54.8g | carbs: 4.2g | net carbs: 3.3g | fiber: 0.9g

17 Caribbean Beef with Peppers

Prep time: 15 minutes | Cook time: 1 hour 5 minutes |
Serves 8

INGREDIENTS:

2 onions, chopped

2 tablespoons avocado oil

2 pounds (907 g) beef stew meat, cubed

2 red bell peppers, seeded and chopped

1 habanero pepper, chopped

4 green chilies, chopped

14.5 ounces (411 g) canned diced tomatoes

2 tablespoons fresh cilantro, chopped

4 garlic cloves, minced

½ cup vegetable broth

Salt and black pepper, to taste

1½ teaspoons cumin

½ cup black olives, chopped

1 teaspoon dried oregano

DIRECTIONS:

Set a pan over medium heat and warm avocado oil.
Brown the beef on all sides; remove and set aside. Stir-
fry in the red bell peppers, green chilies, oregano,
garlic, habanero pepper, onions, and cumin, for about
5-6 minutes. Pour in the tomatoes and broth, and cook
for 1 hour. Stir in the olives, adjust the seasonings and
serve in bowls sprinkled with fresh cilantro.

NUTRITION:

calories: 304 | fat: 14.1g | protein: 25.1g | carbs: 10.9g |
net carbs: 7.9g | fiber: 3.0g

18 Veal with Ham and Sauerkraut

Prep time: 15 minutes | Cook time: 55 minutes | Serves 4

INGREDIENTS:

1 pound (454 g) veal, cut into cubes

18 ounces (510 g) sauerkraut, rinsed and drained

Salt and black pepper, to taste

½ cup ham, chopped

1 onion, chopped

2 garlic cloves, minced

1 tablespoon butter

½ cup Parmesan cheese, grated

½ cup sour cream

DIRECTIONS:

Heat a pot with the butter over medium heat, add in the onion, and cook for 3 minutes. Stir in garlic, and cook for 1 minute. Place in the veal and ham, and cook until slightly browned. Place in the sauerkraut, and cook until the meat becomes tender, about 30 minutes. Stir in sour cream, pepper, and salt. Top with Parmesan cheese and bake for 20 minutes at 350°F (180°C).

NUTRITION:

calories: 431 | fat: 26.9g | protein: 28.6g | carbs: 10.1g | net carbs: 5.9g | fiber: 4.2g

19 Pepperoni and Beef Pizza Meatloaf

Prep time: 10 minutes | Cook time: 60 minutes |
Serves 8

INGREDIENTS:

2 pounds (907 g) ground beef (80/20)

⅓ cup superfine blanched almond flour

¼ cup grated Parmesan cheese

1 tablespoon dried parsley

1 tablespoon dried onion flakes

1 teaspoon kosher salt

½ teaspoon dried oregano leaves

½ teaspoon garlic powder

½ teaspoon ground black pepper

2 large eggs

1 cup marinara sauce, store-bought or homemade, plus more for serving if desired

2 cups shredded whole-milk Mozzarella cheese

4 ounces (113 g) thinly sliced pepperoni

Chopped fresh parsley, for garnish (optional)

DIRECTIONS:

Preheat the oven to 375°F (190°C). Line a 9 by 5-inch loaf pan with foil, leaving 2 inches of foil folded over the outside edges of the pan. The extra foil will make it easier to lift the cooked meatloaf out of the pan.

Place the ground beef, almond flour, Parmesan cheese, parsley, onion flakes, salt, oregano, garlic powder, pepper, and eggs in a large bowl and mix well by hand until the texture is uniform.

Press the meatloaf mixture into the prepared loaf pan and flatten it out. Spoon the marinara evenly over the top and then sprinkle with the Mozzarella cheese. Layer the pepperoni slices on top. Bake, uncovered, for 1 hour, or until a meat thermometer inserted in the center reads 165°F (74°C).

Remove the meatloaf from the oven and let cool for at least 10 minutes in the pan to allow it to firm up before slicing.

Carefully remove the meatloaf from the pan using the foil as handles. Place on a cutting board and remove the foil. You can then cut it into slices and serve on individual plates, or, to dress it up a bit, spread some warm marinara sauce on the bottom of a serving platter, then place the loaf on top of the sauce and garnish with fresh parsley, as shown.

NUTRITION:

calories: 440 | fat: 30.9g | protein: 32.8g | carbs: 3.4g | net carbs: 2.4g | fiber: 1.0g

20 Beef Chuck Roast with Mushrooms

Prep time: 15 minutes | Cook time: 3 hours 10 minutes | Serves 6

INGREDIENTS:

2 pounds (907 g) beef chuck roast, cubed

2 tablespoons olive oil

14.5 ounces (411 g) canned diced tomatoes

2 carrots, chopped

Salt and black pepper, to taste

½ pound (227 g) mushrooms, sliced

2 celery stalks, chopped

2 yellow onions, chopped

1 cup beef stock

1 tablespoon fresh thyme, chopped

½ teaspoon dry mustard

3 tablespoons almond flour

DIRECTIONS:

Set an ovenproof pot over medium heat, warm olive oil and brown the beef on each side for a few minutes. Stir in the tomatoes, onions, salt, pepper, mustard, carrots, mushrooms, celery, and stock.

In a bowl, combine 1 cup water with flour. Place this to the pot, stir then set in the oven, and bake for 3 hours at 325°F (163°C) stirring at intervals of 30 minutes. Scatter the fresh thyme over and serve warm.

NUTRITION: calories: 326 | fat: 18.1g | protein: 28.1g | carbs: 10.4g | net carbs: 6.9g | fiber: 3.5g

Chapter 5. Lamb

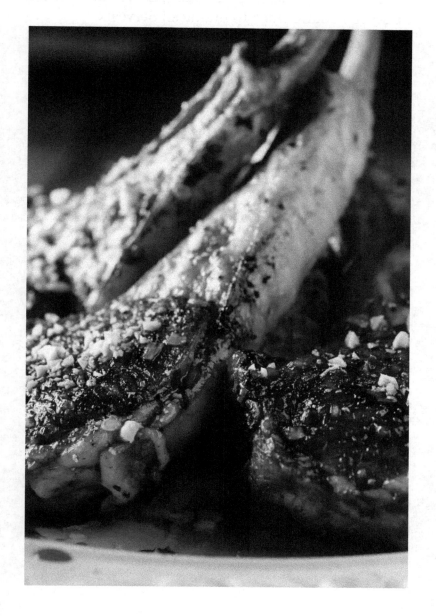

21 White Wine Lamb Chops

Ready in about: 1 hour 10 minutes | Serves: 6

INGREDIENTS:

6 lamb chops

½ tsp sage

½ tsp thyme

1 onion, sliced

3 garlic cloves, minced

2 tbsp olive oil

½ cup white wine

Salt and black pepper to taste

DIRECTIONS:

Heat the olive oil in a pan. Add onion and garlic and cook for 3 minutes until soft. Rub the sage and thyme over the lamb chops. Cook it in the pan for about 3 minutes per side. Set aside.

Pour the white wine and 1 cup of water into the pan and bring the mixture to a boil. Cook until the liquid is reduced by half, about 5 minutes. Add in the chops, reduce the heat, and let simmer for 1 hour. Serve.

NUTRITION: Cal 397, Fat: 30g, Net Carbs: 4.3g, Protein: 16g

22 Oven-Roasted Lamb Chops with Fragrant Curry Sauce

Total time: 45 min; Servings: 4

INGREDIENTS:

2 ribs or French lamb (2 lbs each)

1 tsp melted butter or olive oil

salt and pepper

1-2 tsp garam masala

Indian curry sauce

1 Tbsp butter (or coconut oil)

1 chopped shallot

3 cloves of garlic, fat, minced and raw meat

1 Tbsp finely chopped ginger

½ tsp turmeric

½ tsp fennel seeds

½ tsp mustard seeds

1 ½ cups of diced tomatoes (about 2 medium tomatoes)

1 can (13 oz) coconut milk

1 tsp dried fenugreek leaves: optional, but delicious!

1 tsp salt

1 tsp brown sugar or honey

Coriander garnish, grilled fennel seeds, Aleppo pepper flakes

DIRECTIONS:

Preheat oven to 425 F.

Cut off the excess fat and dry the lamb. Brush with melted butter or olive oil.

Sprinkle both sides with salt, pepper, garam masala and spice mixture (or use Indian Curry powder) and place on a baking sheet and set aside.

Prepare the sauce. Heat the ghee in a large saucepan with medium-sized jumps of gold over medium heat.

Add the shallots, garlic, and ginger and stir for about 3-4 min until golden.

Add diced tomatoes and juices. Continue cooking and stirring for another 5 min until the tomatoes break a little.

Stir, taste, adjust the salt.

Add turmeric, fennel seeds, and mustard seeds and continue to stir for 1 minute.

Place the lamb in the hot oven, roast for 10 min, turn it over, cook for 10 min and turn it for a few minutes if you like a crispy crust.

Be careful not to burn while roasting.

Add coconut milk, fenugreek leaves, salt, and sugar.

Remove the lamb from the oven. Let rest for 5-10 min, then cut the fenugreek sauce and place it on top.

Sprinkle with fresh coriander, grilled fennel seeds (optional), and chili flakes (sweet Aleppo pepper) if you wish.

NUTRITION: Cal 596, Fat: 46g, Net Carbs: 11g, Protein: 37g

23 Grilled Lamb Chops with Dijon Basil Butter

Prep time:20 min; Servings: 4-6

INGREDIENTS:

4 to 6 lamb chops are cut in the center, depending on size

1 Tbsp olive oil

½ tsp garlic powder

1 Tbsp chopped fresh basil

1 garlic clove, finely chopped

1 tsp Dijon mustard

2 Tbsp soft butter

DIRECTIONS:

Sprinkle with garlic powder, sprinkle with oil and let stand until ready to cook.

Grill medium to high for 2 to 5 min per side.

If you think they can be close, remove 1, cut in the middle, and reach the top. You can always put them back in the cook; you cannot undo them ...

When done, remove from heat, divide the basil butter on each heel and serve.

Dijon basil butter:

Put garlic and basil in a small bowl, add mustard and butter and mix well. This can be done in advance, by recording, cooling, and cutting before placing the chops.

NUTRITION: Cal 295 Fat: 20g, Net Carbs: 5g, Protein: 31g

24 Lamb Chops with Tapenade

Preparation Time: 15 minutes

Cooking Time: 25 minutes

Servings: 4

INGREDIENTS:

FOR THE TAPENADE

1 cup pitted Kalamata olive

2 tablespoons chopped fresh parsley

2 tablespoons extra-virgin olive oil

2 teaspoons minced garlic

2 teaspoons freshly squeezed lemon juice

FOR THE LAMB CHOPS

2 (1-pound) racks French-cut lamb chops (8 bones each)

Sea salt

Freshly ground black pepper

1 tablespoon olive oil

DIRECTIONS:

TO MAKE THE TAPENADE

Place the olives, parsley, olive oil, garlic, and lemon juice in a food processor and process until the mixture is puréed but still slightly chunky.

Transfer the tapenade to a container and store it sealed in the refrigerator until needed.

TO MAKE THE LAMB CHOPS

Preheat the oven to 450°F.

Season the lamb racks with pepper and salt

Heat oil

Pan sear the lamb racks on all sides until browned, about 5 minutes in total.

Arrange the racks upright in the skillet, with the bones interlaced, and roast them for about 20 minutes for medium-rare or until the internal temperature reaches 125°F.

NUTRITION: Calories: 387 Fat: 17.4g Fiber: 12.1g Carbohydrates:5.4 g Protein: 18.9g

25 Lamb Lollipops with Garlic And Rosemary

Prep time:10 min; Servings: 4

INGREDIENTS:

8 lamb suckers

2 garlic cloves, finely chopped

2-3 Tbsp olive oil

2-3 sprigs fresh rosemary, removed from the sprig

salt and pepper to taste

DIRECTIONS:

Season each side of the lamb generously with salt and pepper.

Sprinkle some rosemary on each side of the shoulder so that it sticks.

Heat olive oil in a cast-iron pan over medium heat.

Add garlic and rosemary to the pan and spread evenly (about 2 Tbsp rosemary removed from the stem).

Add lamb and brown 4 to 5 min per side.

NUTRITION: Cal 259 Fat: 12.6g, Net Carbs: 4.4g, Protein: 31g

Chapter 6. Pork Recipes

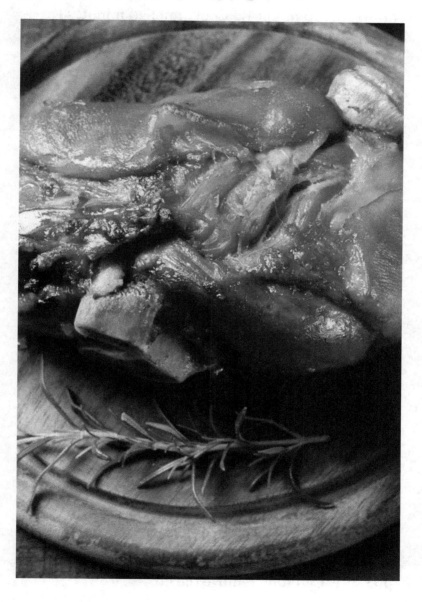

26 Pork and Green Salad

Prep time: 10 minutes | Cook time: 30 minutes | Serves 4

INGREDIENTS:

1 pound (454 g) pork loin roast

½ cup chicken vegetable broth

½ cup water

½ head cabbage, shredded

1 cup baby spinach

1 cup arugula

2 celery with leaves, chopped

4 spring onions, chopped

1 red chili, deseeded and finely chopped

1 teaspoon keto-friendly Thai fish sauce

2 teaspoons coconut aminos

2 teaspoons each sesame oil

Juice of 1 lemon

DIRECTIONS:

Add pork loin roast, vegetable broth and water to the Instant Pot greased with cooking spray.

Secure the lid. Choose the Meat/Stew mode and set cooking time for 30 minutes at High pressure.

Once cooking is complete, use a natural pressure release for 15 minutes, the release any remaining pressure. Carefully remove the lid.

Allow the pork loin roast to cool completely. Shred the meat and transfer to a salad bowl.

Add the cabbage, spinach, arugula, celery, spring onions, and chili.

Make the dressing by mixing the Thai fish sauce, coconut aminos, sesame oil, and lemon juice. Whisk to combine well and dress the salad.

Serve chilled.

NUTRITION:

calories: 279 | fat: 12.7g | protein: 32.5g | carbs: 8.5g | net carbs: 3.9g | fiber: 4.7g

27 Cayenne Pork Saag

Prep time: 10 minutes | Cook time: 20 minutes |
Serves 4

INGREDIENTS:

⅓ cup half-and-half

2 teaspoons garam masala

1 teaspoon minced garlic

1 teaspoon minced fresh ginger

½ teaspoon ground turmeric

½ teaspoon cayenne

1 teaspoon salt

1 pound (454 g) pork shoulder, cut into bite-size cubes

For the Pork Saag:

1 tablespoon peanut oil

1 tablespoon unsweetened tomato purée

¾ cup water

5 ounces (142 g) baby spinach, chopped

Salt, to taste

DIRECTIONS:

In a large bowl, mix the half-and-half, garam masala, garlic, ginger, turmeric, cayenne, and salt. Add the pork and stir to coat.

Marinate the pork for at least 30 minutes in the refrigerator.

Preheat the Instant Pot on Sauté mode. Add the peanut oil and heat until shimmering.

Add the pork with the marinade, and the tomato purée. Cook for 5 to 10 minutes, or until the pork is lightly seared and the tomato purée has been well incorporated. Pour in the water.

Lock the lid. Select Manual mode. Set cooking time for 10 minutes on High Pressure.

When cooking is complete, quick release the pressure. Carefully remove the lid and add the spinach. Mix well to incorporate.

Lock the lid. Select Manual mode. Set cooking time for 2 minutes on High Pressure.

When timer beeps, allow the pressure to release naturally for 5 minutes, then release any remaining pressure. Unlock the lid.

Sprinkle with salt and mix to serve.

NUTRITION:

calories: 335 | fat: 24.0g | protein: 24.0g | carbs: 7.0g | net carbs: 4.0g | fiber: 3.0g

28 Pork Bacon with Mixed Greens

Prep time: 10 minutes | Cook time: 7 minutes |
Serves 2

INGREDIENTS:

7 ounces (198 g) mixed greens

8 thick slices pork bacon

2 shallots, peeled and diced

Nonstick cooking spray

DIRECTIONS:

Begin by preheating the air fryer to 345°F (174°C).

Now, add the shallot and bacon to the Air Fryer cooking basket; set the timer for 2 minutes. Spritz with a nonstick cooking spray.

After that, pause the Air Fryer; throw in the mixed greens; give it a good stir and cook an additional 5 minutes. Serve warm.

NUTRITION:

calories: 259 | fat: 16g | protein: 19g | carbs: 10g | net carbs: 5g | fiber: 5g

29 Pork Cutlets with Mushroom Sauce

Prep time: 10 minutes | Cook time: 15 minutes | Serves 4

INGREDIENTS:

2 teaspoons olive oil

4 pork cutlets

Seasoned salt, to taste

½ teaspoon ground black pepper

½ teaspoon cayenne pepper

1 cup porcini mushrooms, thinly sliced

½ cup scallions, chopped

1 teaspoon roasted garlic paste

1 bay leaf

1 cup chicken vegetable broth

1 tablespoon arrowroot powder

1 tablespoon water

½ cup heavy cream

DIRECTIONS:

Press the Sauté button to heat up the Instant Pot; add the olive oil.

Sear the pork cutlets for 5 minutes or until browned on both sides. Season with salt, black pepper, and cayenne pepper.

Add the mushrooms, scallions, garlic paste, bay leaf, and vegetable broth to the Instant Pot.

Secure the lid. Choose the Manual mode and set cooking time for 10 minutes on High pressure.

Once cooking is complete, use a quick pressure release. Carefully remove the lid.

Whisk the arrowroot powder with water in a small mixing bowl to make the slurry. Ad the slurry with heavy cream to the cooking liquid.

Press the Sauté button to bring the cooking liquid to a boil. Serve the sauce over pork cutlets.

NUTRITION:

calories: 412 | fat: 25.4g | protein: 41.5g | carbs: 2.1g | net carbs: 0.8g | fiber: 1.3g

30 Pork Shank with Radish

Prep time: 15 minutes | Cook time: 44 minutes | Serves 6

INGREDIENTS:

1½ pounds (680 g) pork shank

Seasoned salt and ground black pepper, to taste

1 tablespoons za'atar

1 tablespoon olive oil

1 medium leek, sliced

1 turnip, chopped

1 radish, chopped

1 celery with leaves, chopped

2 garlic cloves, smashed

1 tablespoon coconut aminos

½ teaspoon mustard powder

1 cup beef bone vegetable broth

1 tablespoon flaxseed meal

1 tablespoon water

DIRECTIONS:b

Season the pork shank with salt and black pepper. Sprinkle with za'atar on all sides.

Press the Sauté button to heat up the Instant Pot. Heat the olive oil. Once hot, sear the pork shank for 3 minute per side. Remove the pork from the pot and reserve. Sauté leeks in the pot for 3 minutes.

Add the turnip, radish, celery with leaves, garlic, coconut aminos, mustard powder, and vegetable broth. Put the pork shank back to the Instant Pot.

Secure the lid. Choose the Meat/Stew mode and set cooking time for 35 minutes on High pressure.

Once cooking is complete, use a natural pressure release for 15 minutes, then release any remaining pressure. Carefully remove the lid. Transfer the pork and vegetables to a platter.

Mix flaxseed meal with water to make the slurry. Add to the Instant Pot. Press the Sauté button again and bring the cooking liquid to a boil.

Serve the pork and vegetables with the thickened cooking liquid.

NUTRITION:

calories: 328 | fat: 18.1g | protein: 30.6g | carbs: 9.0g | net carbs: 2.6g | fiber: 6.4g

Chapter 7. Fish and Seafood

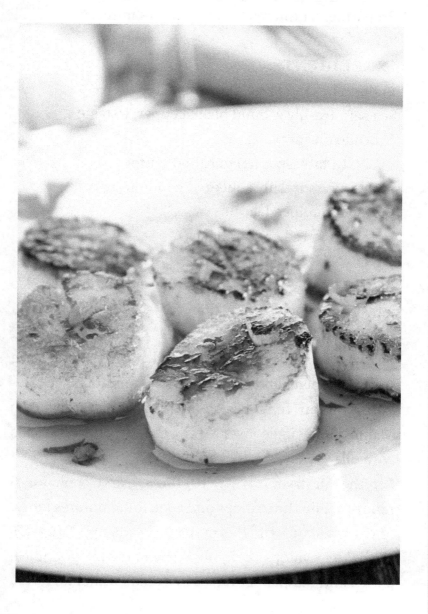

31   Lemon Butter Scallops

Prep time: 5 minutes | Cook time: 15 minutes |
Serves 4

INGREDIENTS:

1 pound (454 g) large sea scallops

Sea salt, freshly ground black pepper, to taste

Avocado oil spray

¼ cup (4 tablespoons) unsalted butter

1 tablespoon freshly squeezed lemon juice

1 teaspoon minced garlic

¼ teaspoon red pepper flakes

DIRECTIONS:

If your scallops still have the adductor muscles attached, remove them. Pat the scallops dry with a paper towel.

Season the scallops with salt and pepper, then place them on a plate and refrigerate for 15 minutes.

Spray the air fryer basket with oil, and arrange the scallops in a single layer. Spray the top of the scallops with oil.

Set the air fryer to 350°F (180°C) and cook for 6 minutes. Flip the scallops and cook for 6 minutes more, until an instant-read thermometer reads 145° F (63°C).

While the scallops cook, place the butter, lemon juice, garlic, and red pepper flakes in a small ramekin.

When the scallops have finished cooking, remove them from the air fryer. Place the ramekin in the air fryer and cook until the butter melts, about 3 minutes. Stir. Toss the scallops with the warm butter and serve.

NUTRITION:

calories: 203 | fat: 12g | protein: 19g | carbs: 3g | net carbs: 3g | fiber: 0g

32 Mackerel with Bell Pepper

Prep time: 15 minutes | Cook time: 20 minutes | Serves 5

INGREDIENTS:

1-pound (454 g) mackerel, trimmed

1 bell pepper, chopped

½ cup spinach, chopped

1 tablespoon avocado oil

1 teaspoon ground black pepper

1 teaspoon keto tomato paste

DIRECTIONS:

In the mixing bowl, mix bell pepper with spinach, ground black pepper, and tomato paste.

Fill the mackerel with spinach mixture.

Then brush the fish with avocado oil and put it in the air fryer.

Cook the fish at 365°F (185°C) for 20 minutes.

NUTRITION:

calories: 252 | fat: 16g | protein: 22g | carbs: 2g | net carbs: 1g | fiber: 1g

33   Dijon Shrimp with Romaine

Prep time: 10 minutes | Cook time: 4 to 6 minutes | Serves 4

INGREDIENTS:

12 ounces (340 g) fresh large shrimp, peeled and deveined

1 tablespoon plus 1 teaspoon freshly squeezed lemon juice, divided

4 tablespoons olive oil or avocado oil, divided

2 garlic cloves, minced, divided

¼ teaspoon sea salt, plus additional to season the marinade

¼ teaspoon freshly ground black pepper, plus additional to season the marinade

⅓ cup sugar-free mayonnaise

2 tablespoons freshly grated Parmesan cheese

1 teaspoon Dijon mustard

1 tinned anchovy, mashed

12 ounces (340 g) romaine hearts, torn

DIRECTIONS:

Place the shrimp in a large bowl. Add 1 tablespoon of lemon juice, 1 tablespoon of olive oil, and 1 minced garlic clove. Season with salt and pepper. Toss well and refrigerate for 15 minutes.

While the shrimp marinates, make the dressing: In a blender, combine the mayonnaise, Parmesan cheese,

Dijon mustard, the remaining 1 teaspoon of lemon juice, the anchovy, the remaining minced garlic clove, ¼ teaspoon of salt, and ¼ teaspoon of pepper. Process until smooth. With the blender running, slowly stream in the remaining 3 tablespoons of oil. Transfer the mixture to a jar; seal and refrigerate until ready to serve.

Remove the shrimp from its marinade and place it in the air fryer basket in a single layer. Set the air fryer to 400°F (205°C) and cook for 2 minutes. Flip the shrimp and cook for 2 to 4 minutes more, until the flesh turns opaque.

Place the romaine in a large bowl and toss with the desired amount of dressing. Top with the shrimp and serve immediately.

NUTRITION:
calories: 329 | fat: 30g | protein: 16g | carbs: 4g | net carbs: 2g | fiber: 2g

34 Cheese Mussel and Tomato Stew

Prep time: 15 minutes | Cook time: 3 minutes |
Serves 6

INGREDIENTS:

1½ pounds (680 g) mussels, scrubbed and debearded

1 cup chicken broth

½ cup dry red wine

2 tablespoons olive oil

2 heaping tablespoons chopped green onions

2 tablespoons chopped fresh coriander

½ teaspoon paprika

½ teaspoon dried marjoram

A pinch ground nutmeg

Sea salt and ground black pepper, to taste

½ (28-ounce / 794-g) can San Marzano tomatoes, crushed

2 cloves garlic, crushed

1 cup shredded Asiago cheese

1 tablespoon chopped fresh dill

1 lemon, sliced

DIRECTIONS:

Combine all the ingredients except the cheese, dill and lemon in the Instant Pot.

Lock the lid. Select the Manual mode and set the cooking time for 3 minutes at Low Pressure.

When the timer beeps, perform a quick pressure release. Carefully remove the lid.

Sprinkle with the cheese and dill. Serve topped with the lemon slices.

NUTRITION:

calories: 298 | fat: 16.7g | protein: 28.1g | carbs: 7.5g | net carbs: 6.7g | fiber: 0.8g

35 Dijon Crab Cake

Prep time: 10 minutes | Cook time: 14 minutes |
Serves 4

INGREDIENTS:

Avocado oil spray

⅓ cup red onion, diced

¼ cup red bell pepper, diced

8 ounces (227 g) lump crab meat, picked over for shells

3 tablespoons finely ground blanched almond flour

1 large egg, beaten

1 tablespoon sugar-free mayonnaise (homemade, here, or store-bought)

2 teaspoons Dijon mustard

⅛ teaspoon cayenne pepper

Sea salt, freshly ground black pepper, to taste

Elevated Tartar Sauce, for serving

Lemon wedges, for serving

DIRECTIONS:

Spray an air fryer–friendly baking pan with oil. Put the onion and red bell pepper in the pan and give them a quick spray with oil. Place the pan in the air fryer basket. Set the air fryer to 400°F (205°C) and cook the vegetables for 7 minutes, until tender.

Transfer the vegetables to a large bowl. Add the crab meat, almond flour, egg, mayonnaise, mustard, and cayenne pepper and season with salt and pepper. Stir until the mixture is well combined.

Form the mixture into four 1-inch-thick cakes. Cover with plastic wrap and refrigerate for 1 hour.

Place the crab cakes in a single layer in the air fryer basket and spray them with oil.

Cook for 4 minutes. Flip the crab cakes and spray with more oil. Cook for 3 minutes more, until the internal temperature of the crab cakes reaches 155°F (68°C).

Serve with tartar sauce and a squeeze of fresh lemon juice.

NUTRITION:

calories: 121 | fat: 8g | protein: 11g | carbs: 3g | net carbs: 2g | fiber: 1g

Chapter 8. Vegetable Recipes

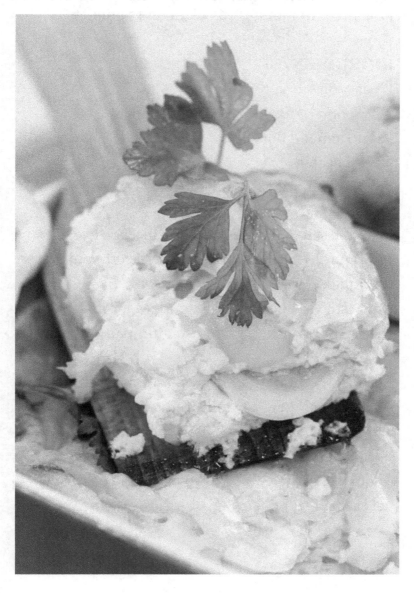

Prep time: 10 minutes | Cook time: 15 minutes | Serves 4

INGREDIENTS:

1 teaspoon sea salt

1 (½-pound / 227-g) zucchini, grated

½ cup almond flour

2 eggs, beaten

1 cup Romano cheese, grated

DIRECTIONS:

Place the salt and grated zucchini in a bowl; let it sit for 15 minutes, squeeze using a cheesecloth and discard the liquid.

Now, stir in the almond flour, eggs, and Romano cheese. Spritz a 12-cup mini-muffin pan with cooking spray.

Bake in the preheated oven for 15 minutes until the surface is no longer wet to the touch. Let them cool about 5 minutes to set up. Bon appétit!

NUTRITION:

calories: 225 | fat: 18.0g | protein: 13.4g | carbs: 3.0g | net carbs: 1.5g | fiber: 1.5g

37 Pumpkin and Cauliflower Curry

Prep time: 15 minutes | Cook time: 7 to 8 hours | Serves 6

INGREDIENTS:

1 tablespoon extra-virgin olive oil

4 cups coconut milk

1 cup diced pumpkin

1 cup cauliflower florets

1 red bell pepper, diced

1 zucchini, diced

1 sweet onion, chopped

2 teaspoons grated fresh ginger

2 teaspoons minced garlic

1 tablespoon curry powder

2 cups shredded spinach

1 avocado, diced, for garnish

DIRECTIONS:

Lightly grease the insert of the slow cooker with the olive oil.

Add the coconut milk, pumpkin, cauliflower, bell pepper, zucchini, onion, ginger, garlic, and curry powder.

Cover and cook on low for 7 to 8 hours.

Stir in the spinach.

Garnish each bowl with a spoonful of avocado and serve.

NUTRITION:

calories: 501 | fat: 44.0g | protein: 7.0g | carbs: 19.0g | net carbs: 9.0g | fiber: 10.0g

38 Garlic Broccoli with Fresh Basil

Prep time: 10 minutes | Cook time: 4 minutes | Serves 4 to 6

INGREDIENTS:

6 cups broccoli florets

1 cup water

1½ tablespoons olive oil

8 garlic cloves, thinly sliced

2 shallots, thinly sliced

½ teaspoon crushed red pepper flakes

Grated zest and juice of 1 medium lemon

½ teaspoon kosher salt

Freshly ground black pepper, to taste

¼ cup chopped roasted almonds

¼ cup finely slivered fresh basil

DIRECTIONS:

Pour the water into the Instant Pot. Place the broccoli florets in a steamer basket and lower into the pot.

Close and secure the lid. Select the Steam setting and set the cooking time for 2 minutes at Low Pressure. Once the timer goes off, use a quick pressure release. Carefully open the lid.

Transfer the broccoli to a large bowl filled with cold water and ice. Once cooled, drain the broccoli and pat dry.

Select the Sauté mode on the Instant Pot and heat the olive oil. Add the garlic to the pot and sauté for 30 seconds, tossing constantly. Add the shallots and pepper flakes to the pot and sauté for 1 minute.

Stir in the cooked broccoli, lemon juice, salt and black pepper. Toss the ingredients together and cook for 1 minute.

Transfer the broccoli to a serving platter and sprinkle with the chopped almonds, lemon zest and basil. Serve immediately.

NUTRITION:

calories: 127 | fat: 8.2g | protein: 5.1g | carbs: 12.2g | net carbs: 10.6g | fiber: 1.6g

39 Cauliflower Egg Bake

Prep time: 10 minutes | Cook time: 25 minutes | Serves 6

INGREDIENTS:

1½ pounds (680 g) cauliflower, broken into small florets

½ cup Greek yogurt

4 eggs, beaten

6 ounces (170 g) ham, diced

1 cup Swiss cheese, preferably freshly grated

DIRECTIONS:

Place the cauliflower into a deep saucepan; cover with water and bring to a boil over high heat; immediately reduce the heat to medium-low.

Let it simmer, covered, approximately 6 minutes. Drain and mash with a potato masher.

Add in the yogurt, eggs and ham; stir until everything is well combined and incorporated.

Scrape the mixture into a lightly greased casserole dish. Top with the grated Swiss cheese and transfer to a preheated at 390°F (199°C) oven.

Bake for 15 to 20 minutes or until cheese bubbles and browns. Bon appétit!

NUTRITION:

calories: 237 | fat: 13.6g | protein: 20.2g | carbs: 7.1g | net carbs: 4.8g | fiber: 2.3g

40 Zucchini Casserole

Prep time: 15 minutes | Cook time: 45 minutes |
Serves 4

INGREDIENTS:

Nonstick cooking spray

2 cups zucchini, thinly sliced

2 tablespoons leeks, sliced

½ teaspoon salt

Freshly ground black pepper, to taste

½ teaspoon dried basil

½ teaspoon dried oregano

½ cup Cheddar cheese, grated

¼ cup heavy cream

4 tablespoons Parmesan cheese, freshly grated

1 tablespoon butter, room temperature

1 teaspoon fresh garlic, minced

DIRECTIONS:

Start by preheating your oven to 370°F (188°C).
Lightly grease a casserole dish with a nonstick cooking
spray.

Place 1 cup of the zucchini slices in the dish; add 1
tablespoon of leeks; sprinkle with salt, pepper, basil,
and oregano. Top with ¼ cup of Cheddar cheese.
Repeat the layers one more time.

In a mixing dish, thoroughly whisk the heavy cream with Parmesan, butter, and garlic. Spread this mixture over the zucchini layer and cheese layers.

Place in the preheated oven and bake for about 40 to 45 minutes until the edges are nicely browned. Sprinkle with chopped chives, if desired. Bon appétit!

NUTRITION:

calories: 156 | fat: 12.8g | protein: 7.5g | carbs: 3.6g | net carbs: 2.8g | fiber: 0.8g

Chapter 9. Soup Recipes

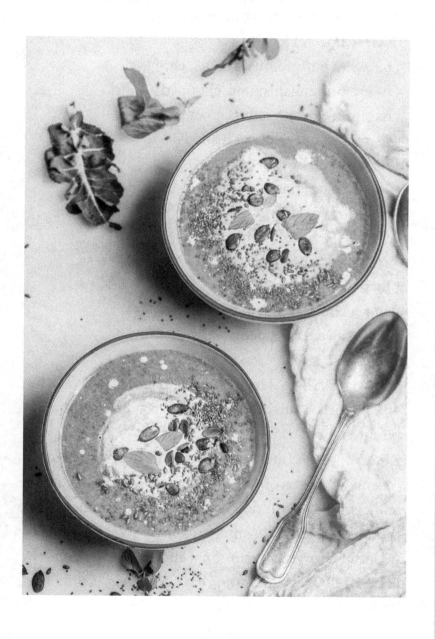

41 Mixed Mushroom Soup

Total Time: approx. 35 minutes|4 servings

INGREDIENTS:

5 oz white button mushrooms, chopped

5 oz cremini mushrooms, chopped

5 oz shiitake mushrooms, chopped

1 vegetable stock cube, crushed

4 oz unsalted butter

1 small onion, finely chopped

1 clove garlic, minced

½ lb celery root, chopped

½ tsp dried rosemary

1 tbsp plain vinegar

1 cup coconut cream

6 leaves basil, chopped

DIRECTIONS:

Melt butter in a saucepan over medium heat. Sauté onion, garlic, mushrooms, and celery until fragrant, 6 minutes.

Reserve some mushrooms for garnishing. Add in rosemary, 4 cups of water, stock cube, and vinegar. Stir and bring to a boil; reduce the heat and simmer for 20 minutes. Mix in coconut cream and puree. Garnish with the reserved mushrooms and basil and serve.

NUTRITION: Cal 506; Fat 46g; Net Carbs 12g; Protein 8g

42 Broccoli & Fennel Soup

Total Time: approx. 25 minutes|4 servings

INGREDIENTS:

1 fennel bulb, chopped

10 oz broccoli, cut into florets

4 cups vegetable stock

Salt and black pepper to taste

1 garlic clove

1 cup cream cheese

2 tbsp butter

½ cup chopped fresh oregano

DIRECTIONS:

Put fennel, broccoli, and garlic in a pot over medium heat and pour in the vegetable stock. Bring to a boil and simmer until the vegetables are soft, about 10 minutes. Season with salt and pepper. Pour in cream cheese, butter, and oregano. Puree the ingredients with an immersion blender until smooth. Serve with cheese crackers.

NUTRITION: Cal 510; Fat 44g; Net Carbs 7g; Protein 16g

43 Keto Reuben Soup

Total Time: approx. 30 minutes |6 servings

INGREDIENTS:

1 onion, diced

7 cups beef stock

1 tsp caraway seeds

2 celery stalks, diced

2 garlic cloves, minced

2 cups heavy cream

1 cup sauerkraut

1 lb corned beef, chopped

3 tbsp butter

1 ½ cups Swiss cheese, grated

Salt and black pepper to taste

DIRECTIONS:

Melt butter in a large pot. Add in onion, garlic, and celery and fry for 3 minutes until tender. Pour the broth over and stir in sauerkraut, salt, caraway seeds, and pepper. Bring to a boil. Reduce the heat to low and add the corned beef. Cook for about 15 minutes. Stir in heavy cream and Swiss cheese and cook for 1 minute. Serve warm.

NUTRITION: Cal 450; Net Carbs 8g; Fat 37g, Protein 23g

44 Effortless Chicken Chili

Total Time: approx. 30 minutes|4 servings

INGREDIENTS:

1 tbsp butter

1 tbsp sesame oil

¼ tsp ginger, ground

4 chicken tenders, cubed

1 onion, chopped

2 cups chicken broth

8 oz diced tomatoes

2 oz tomato paste

1 tbsp cumin

1 red chili pepper, minced

½ cup shredded cheddar

Salt and black pepper to taste

DIRECTIONS:

Put a saucepan over medium heat and add chicken. Cover with water and bring to a boil. Cook for 15 minutes. Transfer to a flat surface to shred with forks. In a pot, warm butter and sesame oil and sauté onion and ginger for 5 minutes. Stir in chicken, tomatoes, cumin, red chili pepper, tomato paste, and chicken broth; season with salt and pepper. Bring the mixture to a boil. Reduce heat and simmer for 10 minutes. Top with cheddar cheese to serve.

NUTRITION: Cal 396; Net Carbs 5.7g; Fat 23g; Protein 38g

45 Parsnip Tomato Soup

Total Time: approx. 40 minutes | 4 servings

INGREDIENTS:

1 tbsp butter

1 tbsp olive oil

1 large red onion, chopped

4 garlic cloves, minced

6 red bell peppers, sliced

1 daikon radish, chopped

2 parsnips, chopped

3 cups chopped tomatoes

4 cups vegetable stock

3 cups coconut milk

2 cups chopped walnuts

1 cup grated Parmesan cheese

DIRECTIONS:

Heat butter and olive oil in a pot over medium heat and sauté onion and garlic for 3 minutes. Stir in bell peppers, daikon radish, and parsnips; cook for 10 minutes. Pour in tomatoes and vegetable stock; simmer for 20 minutes. Puree the soup with an immersion blender. Mix in coconut milk. Garnish with walnuts and Parmesan cheese to serve.

NUTRITION: Cal 955; Net Carbs 4g; Fat 86g, Protein 19.1g

Chapter 10. Dessert Recipes

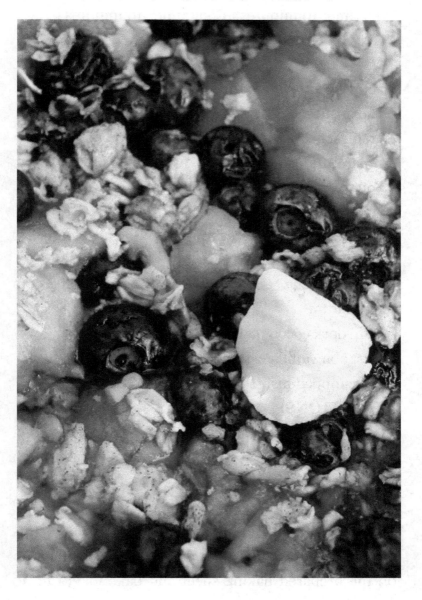

46 Bacon Fudge

Prep time: 10 minutes | Cook time: 40 minutes | Makes 24 bars

INGREDIENTS:

½ cup granulated erythritol–monk fruit blend

6 bacon slices

8 tablespoons (1 stick) unsalted butter, at room temperature

4 ounces (113 g) unsweetened baking chocolate, coarsely chopped

1 cup confectioners' erythritol–monk fruit blend; less sweet: ½ cup

8 ounces (227 g) full-fat cream cheese, at room temperature

¼ cup dark cocoa powder

1 teaspoon vanilla extract

1 cup chopped pistachios

DIRECTIONS:

Preheat the oven to 350°F (180°C). Line the baking sheet with aluminum foil. Line the baking pan with parchment paper and set aside.

In the shallow mixing bowl, put the granulated erythritol–monk fruit blend and dip the bacon slices into it to evenly coat both sides. Place the coated bacon on the prepared baking sheet and bake for 30 to 40 minutes, or until fully cooked. Once cooled, break into smaller pieces and set aside.

In the small microwave-safe bowl, melt the butter and baking chocolate in the microwave in 30-second intervals, then set aside.

In the medium mixing bowl, using an electric mixer on medium high, mix the confectioners' erythritol–monk fruit blend, cream cheese, dark cocoa powder, and vanilla until well combined, stopping and scraping the bowl once or twice, as needed. Add the melted chocolate mixture and combine until fully incorporated. Fold in three-quarters of the candied bacon and the chopped pistachios.

Spread the batter into the prepared baking pan. Sprinkle the remaining candied bacon on top of the fudge.

Put the baking pan in the freezer for about 30 minutes or until the fudge firms. Cut the fudge into 24 squares and serve.

Store the fudge in the refrigerator for up to 5 days or freeze for up to 3 weeks.

NUTRITION: (1 Piece)

Cal: 142 | fat: 13.0g | protein: 3.0g | carbs: 4.0g | net carbs: 2.0g | fiber: 2.0g

47 Blueberry Crisp

Preparation Time: 15 minutes
Cooking Time: 20 minutes
Servings: 2

INGREDIENTS:

1/8 cup almond flour

1 cup fresh blueberries

2 tablespoons powdered swerve sweetener, divided

1/4 cup pecan halves

1 tablespoon ground flax

1/4 teaspoon salt

1/2 teaspoon ground cinnamon

1/2 teaspoon vanilla extract, unsweetened

2 tablespoons unsalted butter

2 tablespoons heavy cream, full-fat

DIRECTIONS:

Preheat oven to 400°F.

Meanwhile, take two ramekins, fill each ramekin with 1/2 cup berries and 1/2 tablespoon sweetener, and stir until combined.

Place remaining ingredients into a food processor, pulse until combined, and then spoon this mixture evenly over berries.

Bake the berries for 15–20 minutes until the topping turns golden-brown and when done, top each with one tablespoon of heavy cream.

Serve straight away.

NUTRITION: Cal: 278 Fat: 11g Fiber: 6.4g Carbohydrates:3.1 g Protein: 6.9g

48 Lemon Coconut Balls

Preparation Time: 40 minutes

Cooking Time: 0 minutes

Servings: 10

INGREDIENTS:

Balls

1/2 cup and 2 tablespoons almond flour

2 teaspoons Truvia

1/16 teaspoon salt

1 tablespoon Splenda sweetener

1/2 of a lemon, zested

1/4 cup cream cheese, full-fat, softened

2 teaspoons lemon juice

1/4 teaspoon vanilla extract, unsweetened

1 teaspoon sour cream, full-fat

Coating

1 teaspoon Truvia

1/4 cup shredded coconut, unsweetened

DIRECTIONS:

Prepare the balls and for this, take a medium-sized bowl, place all of its ingredients in it, and then stir well until the thick dough comes together.

Let the dough chill for 7 minutes.

Meanwhile, take a small bowl, place the coconut in it, add Truvia, and stir until mixed.

After 7 minutes, shape the dough into ten balls of even size and then roll them into coconut until well coated. Arrange balls on a plate, freeze for a minimum of 30 minutes, and serve.

NUTRITION: Cal: 89 Fat: 6.1g Fiber:4.2 g Carbohydrates: 2.1g Protein: 4.1g

49 Almond Shortbread Cookies

Preparation Time: 15 minutes

Cooking Time: 12 minutes

Servings: 6

INGREDIENTS:

1/3 cup coconut flour

1/4 cup erythritol

2/3 cup almond flour

8 drops stevia

1/2 cup butter

1 tsp. almond or vanilla extract

1/4 tsp.. baking powder

For glaze:

1/4 cup coconut butter

8 drops stevia

DIRECTIONS:

In a bowl, add coconut flour, almond flour, erythritol, baking powder, and add vanilla or almond extract, stevia, and melted butter and make a soft dough.

The dough must be divided into two and chill in the refrigerator for 10 minutes.

Roll the dough on a sheet and cut cookies with the help of a cookie cutter.

Place cookies into a baking pan and bake for 6 minutes in a preheated oven at 180C.

Now let the cookies completely cool and apply the glaze.

NUTRITION: Cal: 245 Fat: 9.4g Fiber: 3.1g Carbohydrates:2.9 g Protein: 1.8g

50 Granny Smith Apple Tart

Preparation Time: 15 minutes

Cooking Time: 25 minutes

Servings: 6

INGREDIENTS:

6 tbsp. butter

2 cups almond flour

1 tsp. cinnamon

1/3 cup sweetener

Filling:

2 cups sliced Granny Smith

1/4 cup butter

1/4 cup sweetener

1/2 tsp. cinnamon

1/2 tsp. lemon juice

Topping:

1/4 tsp. cinnamon

2 tbsp. sweetener

DIRECTIONS:

Preheat oven to 370°F and combine all crust ingredients in a bowl.

Press this mixture into the bottom of a greased pan. Bake for 5 minutes.

Meanwhile, combine the apples and lemon juice in a bowl and sit until the crust is ready.

Arrange them on top of the crust.

Combine remaining filling ingredients, and brush this mixture over the apples. Bake for about 30 minutes.

Press the apples down with a spatula, return to oven, and bake for 20 more minutes. Combine the cinnamon and sweetener in a bowl, and sprinkle over the tart.

NUTRITION: Cal: 276 Fat: 11g Fiber: 10.4g Carbohydrates:2.1 g Protein: 3.1g